THE 10-STEP METHOD

TO PREVENT ELDERLY FALLS

(A Case Study Guide Using Fall Prevention Strategies In

Nursing Homes And Assisted Living Facilities)

DR. MICHAEL T. MAGHARI PT, DPT, CES, PTRP, CPAHA

DISCLAIMER AND COPYRIGHT

This book is written for information purposes only, and it is not intended to discourage or replace medical advice. It is not meant to be a substitute for a personal interview with a physician, healthcare professional or provider, and the author is not held liable for any interpretation, use or misuse of the contents hereby presented.

All the intellectual property rights of this book are the property of the author, and by reading its contents, you agree not to republish, distribute, duplicate, reproduce or sell this material to a third party without the express authorization and written consent of the author.

Copyright © 2019

DEDICATION

I dedicate this book to my family, friends, colleagues, patients, and most of all to God who inspires me and gives me the strength. without Him, I can do nothing. To God be The Glory!

TABLE OF CONTENTS

ABSTRACT

Background and purpose: Fall among the elderly populations are a major cause of concern in skilled nursing settings and nursing home facilities. Nursing home falls may result in disability, functional decline, reduced independence, and decreased quality of life in the elderly. In addition, they may have the potential to cause financial burden to family and institution. An effective fall prevention and reduction program is needed to address the problem.

Case description: The fall prevention program has a 10 step-method that will be implemented in any skilled nursing, assisted living, or nursing home facility. It requires an interdisciplinary or multidisciplinary effort between healthcare providers and workers to achieve a common goal. It is important to use evidence-based fall risk assessment tools and a thorough look at the whole person for assessment of fall risks. These 10 steps will be discussed in detail and implemented in the facility to prevent falls.

Outcomes: Measured outcomes will be based on the number of falls per patient that occur daily, fall reoccurrence, and if there are injuries sustained. Functional assessment tools that target muscle strength, endurance, balance, and mobility will be used to measure the progress of the patient and as a baseline for fall risk reduction.

Discussion: Communication between healthcare providers and staff, commitment to improved health outcomes, and consistent implementation and improvement of the fall prevention tasks are key to success in promoting this evidence-based practice. Barriers to success are poor communication, resistance to change, lack of education, and manpower shortages.

BACKGROUND AND PURPOSE

Falls in the elderly are a major source of problems for institutions such as nursing homes and assisted living facilities. According to the U.S. Centers for Disease Control and Prevention or CDC, "It is estimated that around 1.5 million adults over the age of 65 are living in nursing homes and there will be approximately 3 million nursing home patients by 2030. Between 10-20% of nursing home falls result in serious injury for the elderly patient."[1] This increases the burden on patients, families, and nursing homes.

Nursing home patients typically fall 2.6 times each year.[2] Because the outcome from falls can have a serious negative impact, developing a value-based fall prevention program will enable more positive outcomes. Twice as many elderly people fall each year in nursing homes as do

---

[1] United States. Centers for Disease Control and Prevention. *Falls in Nursing Homes*. Centers for Disease Control and Prevention, 2012.
Web. http://www.cdc.gov/HomeandRecreationalSafety/Falls/nursing.html.

[2] Rubenstein LZ, Robbins AS, Josephson KR, Schulman BL, Osterweil D. The value of assessing falls in an elderly population. A randomized clinical trial. *Ann Intern Med.* 1990;113(4):308-316.

in the community; falls occur in 50 to 75% of nursing home patients.[3]

Approximately 5% of seniors age 65 and older reside in a nursing home, and 20% of deaths in nursing home patients may be attributed to falls.[4] These falls have a significant impact on the operation of the nursing home since 2 to 6% of patients who fall end up with a fracture.[5,6] Therefore, the nursing home is the appropriate setting for a program to reduce falls and fractures. One study estimated that 1,800 elderly patients die each year from nursing home falls.[7]

The risk factors that lead to falls may be categorized as intrinsic, extrinsic, and behavioral. In a study performed by Boelens et al., intrinsic factors were defined as muscle strength, balance, reactive power, dual tasking, and sleep

---

[3] Rubenstein LZ. Preventing falls in the nursing home. *Journal of the American Medical Association*. 1997;278(7):595–6.

[4] Rubenstein LZ, Josephson KR, Robbins AS. Falls in the nursing home. *Ann Intern Med*. 1994;121(6):442-451.

[5] Thapa PB, Brockman KG, Gideon P, Fought RL, Ray WA. Injurious falls in non-ambulatory nursing home residents: a comparative study of circumstances, incidence and risk factors. *Journal of the American Geriatrics Society*. 1996; 44:273–8.

[6] Girman, C., J. Chandler, S. Zimmerman, A. Martin, W. Hawkes, J. Hebel, P. Sloane, and J. Magazine. United States. National Library of Medicine. *Prediction of fracture in nursing home residents*. PubMed Health, 2002. Web.

[7] Rubenstein LZ, Robbins AS, Schulman BL, Rosado J, Osterweil D, Josephson KR. Falls and instability in the elderly. *J Am Geriatr Soc*. 1988;36(3):266-278.

disturbance.[8] Static factors involve age, orthostatic hypotension, osteoarthritis, impaired vision, incontinence, mental problems, medical conditions and medications.[8] Medications that increase fall risk in the elderly are categorized into 3 types: a.) CNS or psychoactive medications such as benzodiazepines, antipsychotics, anticonvulsants/mood stabilizers, antidepressants, opioid narcotics/analgesics, anticholinergics/sedatives[9,10]; b.) medications that affect blood pressure or causes hypotension such as beta-blockers/alpha-blockers, calcium channel blockers, antiarrhythmics and diuretics[11, 12,13]; c.) medications that lower blood sugar or antidiabetic drugs such as insulin, sulfonylureas, and meglitinides.[14,15] These

---

[8] Boelens C, Hekman EE, Verkerke GJ. Risk factors for falls of older citizens. Technol Health Care. 2013;21(5):521-33. doi: 10.3233/THC-130748.

[9] Campbell AJ, Robertson MC, Gardner MM, Norton RN, Buchner DM. Psychotropic medication withdrawal and a home-based exercise program to prevent falls: a randomized, controlled trial. J Am Geriatr Soc 1999; 47: 850–3

[10] Darowski A, Chambers SCF and Chambers DJ. Antidepressants and falls. Drugs and Aging 2009 26 (5) 381-394

[11] Darowski A and Whiting R. Cardiovascular drugs and falls. Reviews in Clinical Gerontology 2011, 21 (2), 170-179

[12] Van der Velde N, van den Meiracker AH, Pols HA, Stricker BH, van der Cammen TJ. Withdrawal of fall-risk-increasing drugs in older persons: effect on tilt-tableTable test outcomes. J Am Geriatr Soc 2007; 55:734–739.

[13] Alsop K, MacMahon M. Withdrawing cardiovascular medications at a syncope clinic. Postgrad MJ 2001; 77:403-5.

[14]Jafari B and Britton ME. Hypoglycaemia in elderly patients with type 2 diabetes mellitus: A review of risk factors, consequences and prevention. Journal of Pharmacy Practice and Research. December 2015;45(4):459-469.

extrinsic factors that exist in nursing home and healthcare facilities can increase the risk of patient falls. Bad lighting, inaccessible windows, mobile objects, improper use of assistive devices, clothing, footwear, and excessive demands are some of the external factors.[16] Changes in living conditions, and time of day, such as the increased incidence of falls that has been shown to occur in the afternoon, may not be changed.[17]

The behaviors that may cause a fall include hurrying, taking risks, physical inactivity, and fear.[18] Walking, transferring followed by standing and lowering are at-risk activities, reports Boelens et al.[19] In current facilities, it is a combination of intrinsic, extrinsic, and behavioral factors that contribute to resident's falls and would benefit from a fall prevention program.

---

[15] Chiba Y, Kimbara Y, Kodera R, Tsuboi Y, Sato K, Tamura Y, Mori S, Ito H, Araki A. Risk factors associated with falls in elderly patients with type 2 diabetes. J Diabetes Complications. 2015 Sep-Oct;29(7):898-902.
[16] Boelens et al.
[17] Ibid.
[18] Ibid.
[19] Ibid.

CASE DESCRIPTION: TARGET SETTING

For a licensed Doctor of Physical Therapy that works in skilled nursing facilities and assisted living facilities, majority, if not all the work involves the elderly population. The sample data gathered from a nursing home facility reveals an average of 265 falls happened per year, with an estimate of 22 falls per month and a total of 50%-60% of those falls requiring hospitalization.

The current falls assessment and intervention is usually conducted by nursing staff upon the admission of the patient. A fall risk evaluation form is also completed at the time. The facility promotes a restraint-free environment and seeks to minimize the use of equipment and devices that are considered restraints. Although, Velcro straps may be used in a wheelchair only if the patient can remove them. Devices that are used with discretion include bed alarms, floor mats, scoop mattresses, and hip protectors.

If a patient does fall, nursing staff will assess the patient for signs of injury before proceeding with intervention. The physician is notified of the fall, and if the injury is severe, the patient is sent to the hospital for further consultation. A fall screen is then submitted by the nursing staff to the rehab department for PT and OT to evaluate the patient in areas of muscle strength, balance, mobility, sensory integrity, pain level, need for adaptive equipment or device, and gait performance.

DEVELOPMENT OF THE PROCESS

The current fall protocol in place will benefit from a comprehensive fall prevention and reduction program. A summary of the fall prevention 10-Step method is found in Table 1. The proposed plan consists of a multidisciplinary and interdisciplinary team approach composed of nurses, certified nursing assistants or CNAs, medical doctors, ophthalmologists, optometrists, physical therapists, occupational therapists, and administration as part of the healthcare staff that fosters teamwork to achieve a common goal. The group will work in a coordinated fashion to implement the fall prevention program.

My proposal will address fall prevention and reduction using a 10-Step Method. These steps are:

1.) The use of evidence-based fall assessment tools for residents in the facility

2.) To provide consistent medication review for patients that are high risks for falls

3.) To have regular eye checkups of residents for visual impairments or deficits

4.) The regular monitoring of resident's blood pressure (BP) for orthostatic/postural hypotension

5.) The proposal for the inclusion of vitamin D supplements to residents

6.) The education of patient and family members regarding height, fit, and proper use of assistive devices

7.) The assessment and provision of adaptive devices, tools, and equipment for fall management and injury prevention

8.) To provide safety and environmental assessment in rooms and bathrooms of fall-risk residents

9.) The implementation and provision of balance, strength training, flexibility, and mobility exercises for fall-risk residents

10.) The education of nurses, CNAs, patients and family members regarding fall prevention strategies

Budget considerations are cost effective and include the purchase of vitamin D supplements, Tai Chi training course for 2 physical therapists and estimated annual labor costs of healthcare workers based on their hourly pay rates. Total cost estimate for the fall prevention and reduction program varies on a yearly basis. A summary of estimated annual costs can be found in Table 1.

As a value-based program, the assessment of its effectiveness will be monitored and analyzed. The value of the program, which is defined as the outcomes relative to the costs, will be used to measure the effectiveness of the program.[20] The fall prevention tasks and program will be evaluated using the value equation where outcomes are measured in terms of all services or activities that are involved in meeting patient needs.[21] This will be a comprehensive measurement of many factors that contribute to a patient maintaining the ability to exercise, balance properly, and remain fall free. Furthermore, the value will be measured over long-term outcomes such as sustainable recovery, the need for ongoing interventions,

---

[20] Porter M. What Is Value in Health Care? The New England Journal of Medicine. 2010;363(26):2477-2481.

[21] Ibid.

and any treatment-related side effects.[22] The fall prevention strategies offer a value proposition which is measurable. According to Porter, outcome measurements will include risk factors or initial medical conditions that require adjusting for.[23] Accurate measurements will include adjustments.

If the fall prevention 10-Step Method is successful, the number of falls that occur in the nursing home will be reduced. A literature review that includes 17 trials on fall prevention in nursing homes revealed that exercise programs reduce the rates of falls and prevent the injuries that result from falls.[24] Additionally, Tai Chi exercises are included for balance training, mobility, endurance, and strength. This study reported an estimated reduction of 37% for all injurious falls, 43% reduction for severe injurious falls, and a 61% reduction for falls resulting in fractures.[25] This proposal posits the same positive outcomes will result from the fall prevention tasks using the 10-Step Method.

---

[22] Ibid.

[23] Ibid.

[24] Darowski A, Chambers SCF and Chambers DJ. Antidepressants and falls. Drugs and Aging 2009 26 (5) 381-394

[25] El-Khoury F, Cassou B, Charles M, and Dargent-Molina P. The effect of fall prevention exercise programmes on fall induced injuries in community dwelling older adults: systematic review and meta-analysis of randomised controlled trials. *BMJ*. 2013; 347:1-13. doi: 10.1136/bmj. f6234.

APPLICATION OF THE PROCESS

The fall prevention program has a 10-Step Method of implementation. The target patients are those who are newly admitted to the facility who will undergo the fall risk assessment tools, long-term residents who are high risk for falls, and those who have fallen or have multiple falls. Residents who are included and implemented into the program are those who scored low (≥ 12 seconds) in the timed up and go test also known as TUG test. For the four-stage balance tests, patients who cannot perform side by side, semi-tandem or tandem in heel to toe stance and cannot hold this stance for at least ten seconds are included in the program. For the 30-second chair stand test, residents who scored below average are included in the program.

The frequency of assessment for long-term residents is every 3 months or 12 weeks. In Table 1, it summarizes the tasks along with the existing state activities, proposed systematic fall prevention activities, team responsible for its application, and increased resources or estimated annual costs. The first step is to perform fall risk assessments of patients mentioned above. Physical assessment tools used to determine gait, strength, and balance deficits are the timed up and go or TUG test, four-stage balance test, and 30-second chair stand test. These tests are the most recent, evidence-supported functional measures for identifying people who are at high risk of falling.[26] Currently, they are not used in the facility. Once implemented, they will be carried out by physical therapists, occupational therapists, and nurses. These healthcare providers will perform the tests with consideration of the patient's condition and situation. These assessments are conducted during admissions of residents in the facility, at the start of PT evaluations, on a weekly basis for progress reports, and at the end of treatment sessions. A summary of estimated annual cost is found in Table 1.

The second fall prevention method is to provide a consistent review of medications used that are considered

---

[26] Lusardi MM, Fritz S, Middleton A, et al. 2017. Determining risk of falls in community dwelling older adults: A systematic review and meta-analysis using posttest probability. Journal of Geriatric Physical Therapy 40(1): 1–36.

fall risk for patients taking the drugs. These medications are of 3 categories: they are medications that affect the CNS or psychoactive medications, medications that affect blood pressure or cause hypotension, and medications that lower blood sugar or antidiabetic drugs. Currently, in the facility, medication reviews are not consistent. The proposed frequency would be to conduct 2 to 3 medication reviews in a year on a regular basis. A summary of estimated annual cost is found in Table 1.

The third step in the program is to have regular eye check-ups for residents to assess visual impairments or deficits and are performed by ophthalmologists or optometrists. Regular check-ups should be conducted every 6 months to 1 year. Seniors with visual impairments and deficits are twice as likely to fall compared to those with good vision.[27] a summary of estimated annual cost is found in Table 1.

The fourth method for fall prevention is to have a regular monitoring of resident's blood pressure (BP) for

---

[27] Crews JE. 2016. Falls Among Persons Aged≥ 65 Years with and Without Severe Vision Impairment—United States, 2014. MMWR. Morbidity and mortality weekly report 65(17): 433–7.

orthostatic hypotension. Postural or orthostatic hypotension is defined as a reduction in systolic blood pressure of ≥ 20 mmHg or in diastolic blood pressure of ≥ 10 mmHg within three minutes of standing. If the patient experiences lightheadedness or dizziness on standing, this is also considered a symptom of postural hypotension and therefore means there is a higher risk of them falling. A summary of estimated annual cost is found in Table 1.

The fifth step in the fall prevention program is to introduce vitamin D supplements as part of the resident's nutrition plan. This will be proposed by the administration to the physicians in charge of implementation. Studies show that vitamin D has beneficial effects on its bone-strengthening properties and reduce injury during falls.[28] The cost to the facility for the inclusion of vitamin D per day (1000 IU for 160 residents is 100 Tablets) x 365 days in one year.

The sixth fall prevention strategy is to provide education to patients and family members regarding the

____

[28] Welmerink DB, Longstreth WT, Lyles MF, et al. Cognition and the risk of hospitalization for serious falls in the elderly: results from the Cardiovascular Health Study. J Gerontol A Biol Med Sci 2010 Nov; 65(11):1242-9

height, fit, and proper use of assistive devices. The goals for the use of assistive devices are to improve independent mobility, reduce disability, delay functional decline, and decrease the burden of care.[29,30] Problems that are identified during the assessment of assistive devices are that more than half are of an incorrect height either too high, poor maintenance including loose rubber caps, tips or hand grips, and poor body posture or use including an incorrect gait pattern, or holding the device on the wrong side.[31,32] These problems result in a 30 to 50 percent drop of patients using them right after receiving the assistive devices.[33] Selection of the appropriate device and education are important to decrease the rate of falls and effectively increase the resident's mobility. Assistive devices that are commonly used are canes, crutches, and walkers. Frequency of regular check-ups of assistive

---

[29] Bateni H, Maki BE. Assistive devices for balance and mobility: benefits, demands, and adverse consequences. *Arch Phys Med Rehabil*. 2005;86(1):134–145.

[30] Faruqui SR, Jaeblon T. Ambulatory assistive devices in orthopaedics: uses and modifications. *J Am Acad Orthop Surg*. 2010;18(1):41–50.

[31] Liu HH. Assessment of rolling walkers used by older adults in senior-living communities. *Geriatr Gerontol Int*. 2009;9(2):124–130.

[32] Liu HH, Eaves J, Wang W, Womack J, Bullock P. Assessment of canes used by older adults in senior living communities. *Arch Gerontol Geriatr*. 2011;52(3):299–303.

[33] Bateni H, Maki BE. Assistive devices for balance and mobility: benefits, demands, and adverse consequences. *Arch Phys Med Rehabil*. 2005;86(1):134–145.

devices and patients with family members education should be conducted every 6 months to 1 year. They are conducted by physical and occupational therapists and a summary of estimated annual cost is found in Table 1.

The seventh fall prevention method is the assessment and provision of adaptive devices, tools, and equipment for falls management and injury prevention. Depending on your location, some facilities are restrain-free facilities and are selective in the use of these devices. The use of non-skid socks, fall mats, bed alarms, Velcro straps are use only if residents can remove them, hip protectors, scoop mattresses, protective headgear or helmet, and floor markers are allowed in the facility.

The assessments are performed by physical and occupational therapists and carried out by nurses and CNAs. A summary of estimated annual cost is found in Table 1.

The next or eighth step in fall prevention strategy is to provide safety and environmental assessment in the rooms and bathrooms of fall risk individuals. A study of falls in residential care centers shows that 75% of falls happen in the rooms and bathrooms, 41% happen during transfers, and 36% during walking.[34] Environmental safety assessment in the rooms and bathrooms are performed by occupational therapists and physical therapists. This includes checking to ensure the call lights are working properly, the correct type of bed used, verifying the presence of grab bars in the bathrooms, the availability of equipment, devices, tools for fall prevention, ensuring resident's areas are uncluttered, and there is a clear path to the bathroom, ensure the lights are good and working properly, assess the floors to verify they are free of spills or watermarks and use signs noting wet surfaces when cleaning to avoid slips and falls. A summary of estimated annual cost is found in Table 1, and these assessments are conducted every 6 months to 1-year period.

The ninth method in the 10-step fall prevention program is the implementation and provision of balance, strength training, flexibility, and mobility exercises for fall risk residents. These are conducted by physical and

---

[34] Rapp K, Becker C, Cameron ID, et al. 2012. Epidemiology of falls in residential aged care: analysis of more than 70,000 falls from residents of bavarian nursing homes. Journal of the American Medical Directors Association 13(2): e1–e6.

occupational therapists. It is mentioned above that exercise programs in nursing homes reduce the rates of falls and prevent the injuries resulting from falls.[35] Seniors with muscle weakness, balance problems, unsteady gait, and mobility restrictions are more likely to fall. Exercises to improve balance and increase muscle strength help reduce the risks of falls in seniors.[36,37] National and International health agencies and organizations like the Centers for Disease Control and Prevention or CDC, National Institute for Health and Care Excellence, American Geriatrics Society, British Geriatrics Society, and the American Physical Therapy Association, all recommend strength and balance exercises for residents to prevent falls.[38,39] Tai chi

---

[35] El-Khoury F, Cassou B, Charles M, and Dargent-Molina P. The effect of fall prevention exercise programmes on fall induced injuries in community dwelling older adults: systematic review and meta-analysis of randomised controlled trials. *BMJ*. 2013; 347:1-13. doi: 10.1136/bmj. f6234.

[36] Gillespie L, Robertson M, Gillespie W, et al. 2012. Interventions for preventing falls in older people living in the community. Cochrane Database of Systematic Reviews 9(CD007146).

[37] Sherrington C, Michaleff ZA, Fairhall N, et al. 2016. Exercise to prevent falls in older adults: an updated systematic review and meta-analysis. British Journal of Sports Medicine 4: online first.

[38] Avin KG, Hanke TA, Kirk-Sanchez N, et al. 2015. Management of falls in community dwelling older adults: clinical guidance statement from the Academy of Geriatric Physical Therapy of the American Physical Therapy Association. Physical Therapy 95(6): 815–34.

[39] Kenny R, Rubenstein L, Tinetti M, et al. 2011. Panel on Prevention of Falls in Older Persons, American Geriatrics Society and British Geriatrics Society: Summary of the Updated American Geriatrics Society/British Geriatrics Society

is one exercise program that combines strength training, flexibility, and balance exercises.[40] Exercise equipment and devices like ankle weights, TheraBand, balance foams, cushions, therapeutic balls, fit balls, wobble boards and discs can be used to challenge, improve balance, and increase muscle strength in lower extremities. To have a successful exercise program for fall prevention requires moderate to high challenge balance training and resistance exercises to strengthen lower extremity muscles [41,42] and should be performed a minimum of 30 mins. to 1 hour up to 3 hours for 3x-5x per week for 10 or more weeks.[43] A summary of estimated annual cost is found in Table 1.

The last but not the least of the 10-step method for fall prevention involves the education of nurses, CNAs,

---

clinical practice guideline for prevention of falls in older persons. Journal of the American Geriatrics Society 59: 148–57.

[40] El-Khoury F, Cassou B, Charles M, and Dargent-Molina P. The effect of fall prevention exercise programmes on fall induced injuries in community dwelling older adults: systematic review and meta-analysis of randomised controlled trials. *BMJ*. 2013; 347:1-13. doi: 10.1136/bmj. f6234.

[41] Gillespie L, Robertson M, Gillespie W, et al. 2012. Interventions for preventing falls in older people living in the community. Cochrane Database of Systematic Reviews 9(CD007146).

[42] Sherrington C, Michaleff ZA, Fairhall N, et al. 2016. Exercise to prevent falls in older adults: an updated systematic review and meta-analysis. British Journal of Sports Medicine 4: online first.

[43] Technical Advisory Group for Community Group Strength and Balance Programmes. 2016. Community Group Strength and Balance Programmes: ACC Commissoned Independent Strength and Balance Technical Advisory Group.

patients, and family members on fall prevention strategies. Education provided with a combination of training and staff feedback has been shown to reduce the rates of falls and injurious falls.[44] Staff should not only focus on protection and prevention but also on safety promotion and well-being of the residents.[45] Mobilization is important for residents in the prevention of complications due to immobility, and it promotes independent functioning. Studies show that about 75% of the time falls occur in rooms or bathrooms, 41% are happening during transfers, and 36% during walking.[46] Education on fall prevention strategies includes performing daily rounds every hour, placing fall risk patients close to nursing stations, adjusting height of bed, closing the gap or distance between wheelchair and bed in standing and transfers, ensuring call lights are easy to reach, making sure wheelchairs are

---

[44] Hill AM, McPhail SM, Waldron N, et al. 2015. Fall rates in hospital rehabilitation units after individualised patient and staff education programmes: a pragmatic, stepped-wedge, cluster-randomised controlled trial. The Lancet 385(9987): 2592–9.

[45] Clancy A, Mahler M. 2016. Nursing staffs' attentiveness to older adults falling in residential care–an interview study. Journal of clinical nursing 25(9–10): 1405–15.

[46] Rapp K, Becker C, Cameron ID, et al. 2012. Epidemiology of falls in residential aged care: analysis of more than 70,000 falls from residents of bavarian nursing homes. Journal of the American Medical Directors Association 13(2): e1–e6.

locked when standing, during transfers, and the use of potty chairs near the bed for incontinent patients. It will be conducted by physical and occupational therapists 3 times or every 4 months in a year. A summary of estimated annual cost is found in Table 1.

OUTCOME

The outcome of the fall prevention program will be determined based on the actual number of falls per calendar year, their reoccurrence, and the severity of falls resulting in injury and hospitalization. As mentioned above, the current data gathered in the facility reveals an average of 265 falls per year, and an estimate of 22 falls per month with 50%-60% of those falls requiring hospitalization. The goal is to reduce the number of falls and reoccurrence by an average of 50% or more within six months to one year using the fall prevention tasks and 10 step method. The falls assessment tools and program are conducted on a regular basis for a 1-year period.

DISCUSSION

The fall prevention program with the 10-step method will achieve its goals through continuous quality improvements. As information is obtained, adjustments can be made, and the program itself improved. Implementing an integrated whole-of-system approach and precautionary measures will succeed in reducing the rate of falls. Secondary analysis will include the financial tracking of cost savings. The nursing home and assisted living facility will experience cost savings and an increase in revenue from this program. Additionally, regulatory and accrediting agencies will rate the nursing home with higher scores after implementation and improved quality performance. There will be challenges and barriers along the way, but consistent implementation and a willingness to change and adapt with a communal mindset to work alongside an interdisciplinary or multidisciplinary team of healthcare providers with patients and their families are worthwhile endeavors that will ultimately improve the quality of life and the functional mobility of nursing home residents.

BIBLIOGRAPHY

Alsop K, MacMahon M. Withdrawing cardiovascular medications at a syncope clinic. Postgrad MJ 2001; 77:403-5.

Avin KG, Hanke TA, Kirk-Sanchez N, et al. 2015. Management of falls in community dwelling older adults: clinical guidance statement from the Academy of Geriatric Physical Therapy of the American Physical Therapy Association. Physical Therapy 95(6): 815–34.

Bateni H, Maki BE. Assistive devices for balance and mobility: benefits, demands, and adverse consequences. *Arch Phys Med Rehabil*. 2005;86(1):134–145.

Boelens C, Hekman EE, Verkerke GJ. Risk factors for falls of older citizens. Technol Health Care. 2013;21(5):521-33. doi: 10.3233/THC-130748.

Campbell AJ, Robertson MC, Gardner MM, Norton RN, Buchner DM. Psychotropic medication withdrawal and a home-based exercise program to prevent falls: a randomized, controlled trial. J Am Geriatr Soc 1999; 47: 850–3

Chiba Y, Kimbara Y, Kodera R, Tsuboi Y, Sato K, Tamura Y, Mori S, Ito H, Araki A. Risk factors associated with falls in elderly patients with type 2 diabetes. J Diabetes Complications. 2015 Sep-Oct;29(7):898-902.

Clancy A, Mahler M. 2016. Nursing staffs' attentiveness to older adults falling in residential care–an interview study. Journal of clinical nursing 25(9–10): 1405–15.

Darowski A, Chambers SCF and Chambers DJ. Antidepressants and falls. Drugs and Aging 2009 26 (5) 381-394

Darowski A and Whiting R. Cardiovascular drugs and falls. Reviews in Clinical Gerontology 2011, 21 (2), 170-179

El-Khoury F, Cassou B, Charles M, and Dargent-Molina P. The effect of fall prevention exercise programmes on fall induced injuries in community dwelling older adults: systematic review and meta-analysis of randomised controlled trials. *BMJ*. 2013; 347:1-13. doi: 10.1136/bmj. f6234.

Faruqui SR, Jaeblon T. Ambulatory assistive devices in orthopaedics: uses and modifications. *J Am Acad Orthop Surg*. 2010;18(1):41–50.

Gillespie L, Robertson M, Gillespie W, et al. 2012. Interventions for preventing falls in older people living in the community. Cochrane Database of Systematic Reviews 9(CD007146).

Girman, C., J. Chandler, S. Zimmerman, A. Martin, W. Hawkes, J. Hebel, P. Sloane, and J. Magazine. United States. National Library of Medicine. *Prediction of fracture in nursing home residents*. PubMed Health, 2002. Web.

Hill AM, McPhail SM, Waldron N, et al. 2015. Fall rates in hospital rehabilitation units after individualised patient and staff education programmes: a pragmatic, stepped-wedge, cluster-randomised controlled trial. The Lancet 385(9987): 2592–9.

Jafari B and Britton ME. Hypoglycaemia in elderly patients with type 2 diabetes mellitus: A review of risk factors, consequences and prevention. Journal of Pharmacy Practice and Research. December 2015;45(4):459-469.

Kenny R, Rubenstein L, Tinetti M, et al. 2011. Panel on Prevention of Falls in Older Persons, American Geriatrics Society and British Geriatrics Society: Summary of the Updated American Geriatrics Society/British Geriatrics Society clinical practice guideline for prevention of falls in older persons. Journal of the American Geriatrics Society 59: 148–57.

Liu HH. Assessment of rolling walkers used by older adults in senior-living communities. *Geriatr Gerontol Int.* 2009;9(2):124–130.

Liu HH, Eaves J, Wang W, Womack J, Bullock P. Assessment of canes used by older adults in senior living communities. *Arch Gerontol Geriatr.* 2011;52(3):299–303.

Lusardi MM, Fritz S, Middleton A, et al. 2017. Determining risk of falls in community dwelling older adults: A systematic review and meta-analysis using posttest probability. Journal of Geriatric Physical Therapy 40(1): 1–36.

Porter M. What Is Value in Health Care? *The New England Journal of Medicine.* 2010;363(26):2477-2481.

Rapp K, Becker C, Cameron ID, et al. 2012. Epidemiology of falls in residential aged care: analysis of more than 70,000 falls from residents of Bavarian nursing homes. Journal of the American Medical Directors Association 13(2): e1–e6.

Rubenstein LZ, Robbins AS, Josephson KR, Schulman BL, Osterweil D. The value of assessing falls in an elderly population. A randomized clinical trial. *Ann Intern Med.* 1990;113(4):308-316.

Rubenstein LZ. Preventing falls in the nursing home. *Journal of the American Medical Association.* 1997;278(7):595–6.

Rubenstein LZ, Josephson KR, Robbins AS. Falls in the nursing home. *Ann Intern Med.* 1994;121(6):442-451.

Rubenstein LZ, Robbins AS, Schulman BL, Rosado J, Osterweil D, Josephson KR. Falls and instability in the elderly. *J Am Geriatr Soc.* 1988;36(3):266-278.

Sherrington C, Michaleff ZA, Fairhall N, et al. 2016. Exercise to prevent falls in older adults: an updated systematic review and meta-analysis. British Journal of Sports Medicine 4: online first.

Technical Advisory Group for Community Group Strength and Balance Programmes. 2016. Community Group Strength and Balance Programmes: ACC Commissoned Independent Strength and Balance Technical Advisory Group.

Thapa PB, Brockman KG, Gideon P, Fought RL, Ray WA. Injurious falls in non-ambulatory nursing home residents: a comparative study of circumstances, incidence and risk factors. *Journal of the American Geriatrics Society.* 1996; 44:273–8.

United States. Centers for Disease Control and Prevention. Falls in Nursing Homes. Centers for Disease Control and Prevention, 2012. Web. http://www.cdc.gov/HomeandRecreationalSafety/Falls/nursing.html.

Van der Velde N, van den Meiracker AH, Pols HA, Stricker BH, van der Cammen TJ. Withdrawal of fall-risk-increasing drugs in older persons: effect on tilt-Table test outcomes. J Am Geriatr Soc 2007; 55:734–739.

Welmerink DB, Longstreth WT, Lyles MF, et al. Cognition and the risk of hospitalization for serious falls in the elderly: results from the Cardiovascular Health Study. *J Gerontol A Biol Med Sci* 2010 Nov; 65(11):1242-9

TABLE: Summary of the 10-Step Method for Fall Prevention

Fall prevention Tasks (The 10-Step Method)	Existing State Activities	Measures, Triggers and Interventions (proposed systematic fall prevention activities)	Interdisciplinary/ Multidisciplinary Team Approach (team members)	Increased Resources (estimated annual cost)
1.) The use of evidence-based falls assessment tools for residents in the facility	none	a.) timed up and go or TUG test - Patients aged 65 years and older who take ≥12 seconds to complete the TUG are at risk of falling. b.) 30 second chair stand test - Please refer to the chart below for reference. c.) four-stage balance test Patients aged 65 years or older who do not progress to the tandem, heel to toe stance or cannot hold this stance for at least ten seconds are at increased risk of falling. Frequency in using the screening tools should start during admissions of residents in the facility, at the start of PT evaluations, on a weekly basis for progress reports and at the end of treatment sessions. Frequency of assessment for long term residents are conducted every 3 months or 12 weeks.	performed by PT, OT and Nurses	The cost can range from the services of PT, OT and nurses if performed beyond regular office hours. extra hours needed would be 1–3 hours. Estimated annual costs are based on PT, OT and Nurse's hourly rates

2.) To provide consistent medication reviews on patients that are high risks for falls	not on a regular basis	a.) CNS or psychoactive medications. Examples are benzodiazepines, antipsychotics, anticonvulsants, mood stabilizers, antidepressants, opioid narcotics, analgesics, anticholinergics, sedatives b.) medications that affects blood pressure or causes hypotension. Examples are beta-blockers, alpha-blockers, calcium channel blockers, antiarrhythmics and diuretics c.) medications that lower blood sugar or antidiabetic agents. Examples are insulin, sulfonylureas and meglitinides Frequency of the medication reviews should be conducted 2 to 3 reviews every year.	performed by MDs or PCPs (primary care physicians), pharmacists	There is no cost involved if medication reviews are performed 2 up to 3 times per year. If it's above, the costs of the physicians or MDs and pharmacists will be on an hourly basis. extra hours needed would be 1-3 hours. Estimated annual costs are based on Physicians and Pharmacist's hourly rates
3.) To have regular eye check-ups on residents for visual impairment or deficits	not on a regular basis	Older people with visual impairments or deficits is twice as likely to fall compared to those with good vision. Frequency for regular eye check-ups should be performed every 6 months to 1-year.	Ophthalmolog ists and Optometrists	If there is a need for the services of an ophthalmologis ts and optometrists beyond the free range of services, they are paid on an hourly basis. Extra hours needed would be 2-3 hours. Estimated annual costs are based on Ophthalmologis ts and Optometrist's hourly rates

4.) The regular monitoring of patient's blood pressure (BP) for orthostatic/ postural hypotension	performed at the start and end of an 8-hour work shift by nurses and CNA's	postural or orthostatic hypotension is defined as a reduction in systolic blood pressure of ≥ 20 mmHg or in diastolic blood pressure of ≥ 10 mmHg within three minutes of standing.[1] If the patient experiences light-headedness or dizziness on standing, this is also considered a symptom of postural hypotension and therefore means there is a higher risk of them falling.	nurses and CNAs	If the work is performed beyond regular office hours. healthcare staff will be paid on an hourly basis. Hours required will be 1-3 hours. Estimated annual costs are based on Nurses and CNA's hourly rates
5.) The proposal for the inclusion of vitamin D supplement to residents	only on MD's or Physicians approval	vitamin D has beneficial effects in its bone strengthening properties and reduce injury during falls.	MDs or PCPs Primary Care Physicians	Estimated cost of vitamin D/day (1000 IU) for 160 residents = 100 Tablets x 365 days/1 year
6.) The education of patients and family members regarding the height, fit and proper use of assistive devices	only when patients and family members request for it	canes - standard, straight, tripod and quad canes. crutches - axillary crutches, forearm or lofstrand and platform crutches. walkers – standard, front wheeled or two wheeled and four wheeled known as rollator walkers. Frequency for regular check-ups of assistive devices and patients with family members education should be conducted every 6 months to 1 year.	PT and OT	If the education is performed beyond regular office hours. healthcare staff will be paid on an hourly basis. Hours required will be 1-3 hours. Estimated annual costs are based on PT and OT hourly rates

7.) The assessment and provision of adaptive devices, tools and equipment for falls management and injury prevention	only when a patient falls and is referred to rehab for screening and assessment	the use of non-skid socks, fall mats, bed alarms, Velcro straps are used only if residents can remove them, hip protectors, scoop mattresses, protective headgears or helmets and floor markers can be used in the facility for fall risk reduction and management. Frequency for regular assessments of tools, adaptive devices and equipment should be conducted every 6 months to 1 year.	conducted by PT and OT, carried out by nurses and CNAs.	If the assessment is performed beyond regular office hours. healthcare staff will be paid on an hourly basis. Hours required will be 1–3 hours. Estimated annual costs are based on PT, OT, Nurses and CNA's hourly rates
8.) To provide safety and environmental assessment in the rooms and bathrooms of fall risk patients	only when a patient falls and is referred to rehab for screening and assessment	call lights are working properly, the type of bed used, presence of grab bars in the bathrooms, availability of equipment, devices, tools for fall prevention, the resident's areas are uncluttered and have a clear path in going to the bathroom, ensure lights are good and working properly, assess floors that they are free from spills or water marks and the use of signs noting wet surfaces when cleaning to avoid slips and falls. Frequency of safety and environmental assessments of rooms and bathrooms should be conducted every 6 months to 1 year.	OT and PT	If the assessment is performed beyond regular office hours. healthcare staff involved will be paid on an hourly basis. Hours required will be 1–3 hours. Estimated annual costs are based on PT and OT hourly rates

9.) The implementation and provision of balance, strength training, flexibility and mobility exercises for fall risk residents	No Tai-chi program in place	Tai-chi exercises are provided to improve balance, muscle strength, promote flexibility and endurance. the use of exercise equipment and tools like ankle weights, TheraBand, balance foams, cushions, therapeutic balls, fit balls, wobble boards, discs can be used to challenge, improve balance and increase muscle strength of lower extremities. A successful and effective exercise program for fall prevention requires the intensity of the program to be moderate to high in challenging balance training and resistance exercises to increase muscle strength. the frequency should be performed for a minimum of 30 mins. To 1 hour and up to 3 hours 3x to 5x per week for 10 or more weeks.	PT and OT	Tai-chi training course for 2 Physical Therapists Estimated cost depends on the tai-chi program chosen
10.) The education of nurses, CNAs, patients and family members regarding fall prevention strategies	none	Fall prevention strategies includes performing daily rounds every hour and place fall risk patients close to nursing stations. adjusting height of bed and closing the gap or distance between wheelchair and bed in standing and transfers, call lights are easy to reach, wheelchairs are locked when standing, during transfers and the use of potty chairs near the bed for incontinent patients. Frequency of implementation is conducted 3 times or every 4 months per year.	PT and OT	If the education is implemented beyond office hours. healthcare staf involved will be paid on an hourly basis. Hours required will be 1-3 hours. Estimated annual costs are based on PT and OT hourly rates